FOCUSING ON YOUR CHILD

All the information you ne ed to know before and afte r giving birth

By

Carol . J. Johnson

Table of contents

Introduction

The main hour after birth impacts the endurance, future wellbeing, and prosperity of a recently conceived newborn child. The wellbeing laborers play a significant part as of now. The consideration they give during this

period is basic in assisting with forestalling entanglements and guaranteeing endurance. All moms need assistance, backing, and exhortation in the underlying few days after conveyance to guarantee legitimate care of their recently conceived child. The four fundamental requirements of ALL children at the hour of birth (and for the initial not many long stretches of life) are: These fundamental necessities demonstrate that a child's endurance is absolutely subject to her mom and other guardians. Subsequently it is essential to promptly give appropriate consideration to every one of the youngsters after birth. All babies require fundamental infant care to limit the gamble of sickness and boost their development and improvement. This care will likewise forestall numerous infant crises. For instance, the umbilical line might be the most widely recognized wellspring of neonatal sepsis and furthermore of lockjaw contamination, and great rope care can emphatically lessen the dangers of these difficult circumstances. Restrictive breastfeeding has a critical defensive impact against contaminations. Early breastfeeding and keeping the child near the mother decrease the gamble of hypothermia and hypoglycemia

Chapter 1

Pre-birth Care

Ladies who suspect they might be pregnant ought to plan a visit to their medical services supplier to start pre-birth care. Pre-birth visits to a medical services supplier for the most part incorporate an actual test, weight checks, and giving a pee test. Contingent upon the phase of the pregnancy, medical services suppliers may likewise blood tests and imaging tests, like ultrasound tests. These visits additionally incorporate conversations about the mother's wellbeing, the hatchling's wellbeing, and any inquiries concerning the pregnancy.

Pre-Pregnancy and pre-birth care can assist with forestalling inconveniences and illuminate ladies about significant advances they can take to safeguard their newborn child and guarantee a sound pregnancy. With customary pre-birth care ladies can Diminish the gamble of pregnancy inconveniences. Following a sound, safe eating regimen; getting customary activity as prompted by a medical services supplier; and keeping away from openness to possibly destructive substances, for example, lead and radiation can assist with diminishing the gamble for issues during pregnancy and advance fetal wellbeing and improvement. Controlling existing circumstances, for example, hypertension and diabetes, is essential to forestall serious inconveniences and their belongings.

Diminish the hatchling's and newborn child's gamble for inconveniences. Tobacco smoke and liquor use during pregnancy have been displayed to expand the gamble for Unexpected Newborn child Passing Syndrome.6 Liquor use likewise builds the gamble for fetal liquor range issues, which can cause different issues like unusual facial highlights, having a little head, unfortunate dexterity, unfortunate memory, scholarly incapacity, and issues with the heart, kidneys, or bones. As indicated by one ongoing review upheld by the NIH, these and other long-haul issues can happen even with low degrees of pre-birth liquor openness. What's more, taking 400 micrograms of folic corrosive day to day diminishes the gamble for brain tube surrenders by 70%.2,9 Most pre-birth nutrients contain the suggested 400 micrograms of folic corrosive as well as different nutrients that pregnant ladies and their creating hatchling need.1,10 Folic corrosive has been added to food varieties like cereals, breads, pasta, and other grain-based food varieties. Albeit a connected structure (called folate) is available in squeezed orange and verdant, green vegetables (like kale and spinach), folate isn't retained as well as folic corrosive. Pre-birth classes in this manner Assist with guaranteeing the drugs ladies take are protected. Ladies shouldn't accept specific prescriptions, including some skin inflammation treatments11 and dietary and home-grown supplements,12 during pregnancy since they can hurt the hatchling.

Picking a pre-birth care focus

Contemplate what you desire to acquire from antenatal classes so you can find the kind of class that suits you best. Places in antenatal classes can get reserved early. It's really smart to begin making enquiries right off the bat in pregnancy so you can get a spot in the class that you pick. You can go to more than 1 class. To learn about classes close to you, ask your maternity specialist, wellbeing guest or GP. NHS antenatal classes are free. Address your local area maternity specialist on the off chance that you can't go to classes.

When to have antenatal classes

You could possibly go to basic classes on child care right off the bat in pregnancy, however most antenatal classes start around 8 to 10 weeks before your child is expected, when you're around 30 to 32 weeks pregnant. On the off chance that you're expecting twins, begin your classes when you're around 24 weeks pregnant in light of the fact that your children are bound to early be conceived. A few units offer extraordinary antenatal classes on the off chance that you're anticipating products - get some information about this.

What occurs in antenatal classes

Classes are typically held one time each week, either during the day or at night, for something like 2 hours. A few classes are for only for you, others invite accomplices or companions to some or the entirety of the meetings. In certain areas, there are set classes for on the off chance that you're single, a young person or on the other hand on the off chance that English isn't your most memorable language.

The sorts of subjects covered by antenatal classes are:

- Wellbeing in pregnancy, including a ssound/healthy eating regimen
- Activities to keep you fit and dynamic during pregnancy
- What occurs during work and birth
- Adapting to work and data about various kinds of relief from discomfort
- Step by step instructions to help yourself during work and birth
- Unwinding procedures
- Data about various types of birth and intercessions, like

forceps or vacuum conveyance

- Really focusing on your child, including taking care of

Your wellbeing after the birth.

Supplemental courses for those who've proactively had a child

Feelings and sentiments during pregnancy, birth and later

A few classes cover this large number of subjects. Others center around specific perspectives, like activities and unwinding, or really focusing on your child.

Nourishment

Eating great is quite possibly of everything thing you can manage during pregnancy. Great nourishment assists you with taking care of the additional requests on your body as your pregnancy advances. The objective is to adjust getting an adequate number of supplements to help the development of your hatchling and keeping a solid weight

A solid eating routine is a significant piece of a sound way of life whenever however is particularly indispensable on the off chance that you're pregnant or arranging a pregnancy. Eating strongly during pregnancy will assist your child with creating and develop.

You don't have to start a new and improved eating routine, however it's essential to eat a wide range of food varieties consistently to get the right equilibrium of supplements that you and your child need.

It's ideal to get nutrients and minerals from the food varieties you eat, however when you're pregnant you really want to take a folic corrosive enhancement too, to ensure you get all that you need. Try to have a solid breakfast consistently, in light of the fact that this can assist you with trying not to nibble on food varieties that are high in fat and sugar. Eating strongly frequently implies changing the measures of various food varieties you eat, with the goal that your eating routine is fluctuated, as opposed to removing every one of your top choices. You don't have to accomplish this offset with each dinner, however, attempt to get the equilibrium directly more than seven days. . A pregnant lady needs more calcium, folic acid, iron and protein. A solid pregnancy diet ought to incorporate bunches of foods grown from the ground, especially during a lady's second and third trimesters. These brilliant food varieties are low in calories and loaded up with fibre, nutrients and minerals Eat a lot of products of the soil because these give nutrients and minerals, as well as fibre, which helps processing and can assist with forestalling obstruction. Eat something like 5 segments of different foods grown from the ground consistently - these can incorporate new, frozen, canned, dried or squeezed. Continuously wash new foods grown from the ground cautiously.

Protein in pregnancy

Eat some protein-rich food varieties consistently. Wellsprings of protein include:

Beans

Beats

Fish

Eggs

Meat (however stay away from liver)

Poultry

Nuts .

Pick lean meat, eliminate the skin from poultry, a do whatever it takes not to add additional fat or oil while cooking meat. Peruse more about eating meat in a solid manner. Ensure poultry, burgers, frankfurters and entire cuts of meat, for example, sheep, hamburger and pork are cooked completely until steaming the whole way through. Make sure that there is no pink meat, and that juices have no pink or red in them. Attempt to eat 2 segments of fish every week, 1 of which ought to be sleek fish like salmon, sardines or mackerel. Learn about the medical advantages of fish and shellfish. There are a few sorts of fish you ought to stay away from when you're pregnant or intending to get pregnant, including shark, swordfish and marlin.

At the point when you're pregnant, you ought to try not to have multiple segments of sleek fish seven days, like salmon, trout, mackerel and herring, since it can contain contaminations (poisons). You ought to try not to eat a few crude or to some degree cooked eggs, as there is a gamble of salmonella.Eggs delivered under the English Lion Code of Training are ok for pregnant ladies to eat crude or to some extent cooked, surprisingly rushes that have been inoculated against salmonella.These eggs have a red lion logo stepped on their shell. Pregnant ladies can eat these crude or to some degree cooked (for instance, delicate bubbled eggs).Eggs that poor person been delivered under the Lion Code are viewed as less protected, and pregnant ladies are encouraged to try not to eat them crude or to some degree cooked, remembering for mousse, mayonnaise and soufflé. These eggs ought to be cooked until the white and the yolk are hard.

Boring food varieties (starches) in pregnancy

Boring food varieties are a significant wellspring of energy, a few nutrients and fiber, and assist you with feeling full without containing an excessive number of calories. They incorporate bread, potatoes, breakfast cereals, rice, pasta, noodles, maize, millet, oats, sweet potatoes and cornmeal. In the event that you are having chips, go for broiler chips lower in fat and salt. These food varieties ought to make up a little more than a third of the food you eat. Rather than refined boring (white) food, pick wholegrain or higher-fibre choices, for example, whole-wheat pasta, earthy coloured rice or essentially leaving the skins on potatoes.

Dairy in pregnancy

Dairy food varieties like milk, cheddar, fromage frais and yogurt are significant in pregnancy since they contain calcium and different supplements that you and your child need. Pick low-fat assortments at every possible opportunity, for example, semi-skimmed, 1% fat or skimmed milk, low-fat and lower-sugar yogurt and diminished fat hard cheddar. On the off chance that you incline toward dairy choices, for example, soya beverages and yoghurts, go for unsweetened, calcium-strengthened adaptations. There are a few cheeses you ought to keep away from in pregnancy, including unpasteurised cheeses.

Supplements

Ask your medical services supplier, Regardless of whether you eat a solid eating routine, you can pass up key supplements. Taking a day to day pre-birth nutrient in a perfect world beginning something like three months before origination can assist with filling any holes. Your medical services supplier could suggest extraordinary enhancements in the event that you follow a severe veggie lover diet or have a persistent medical issue.

Work out

Converse with your medical services supplier about practicing during pregnancy. For most pregnant ladies, practicing is protected and smart for yourself as well as your child. On the off chance that you and your pregnancy are solid, practice won't expand your gamble of having an unsuccessful labor (when a child kicks the bucket in the belly before 20 weeks of pregnancy), an untimely child (brought into the world before 37 weeks of pregnancy) or a child brought into the world with low birthweight (under 5 pounds)

Practice DURING PREGNANCY

At your most memorable pre-birth care exam, ask your medical services supplier whether practice during pregnancy is alright for you. Sound pregnant ladies need somewhere around 2½ long stretches of oxygen consuming movement, like strolling or swimming, every week. Customary active work can assist with diminishing your gamble of pregnancy inconveniences and straightforwardness pregnancy distresses, like back torment. A few exercises, for example, b-ball, hot yoga, downhill skiing, horseback riding and scuba plunging, aren't protected during pregnancy.

Is it protected to practice during pregnancy?

Converse with your medical services supplier about practicing during pregnancy. For most pregnant ladies, practicing is protected and smart for yourself as well as your child. On the off chance that you and your pregnancy are sound, practice won't expand your gamble of having an unsuccessful labor (when a child kicks the bucket in the belly before 20 weeks of pregnancy), an untimely child (brought into the world before 37 weeks of pregnancy) or a child brought into the world with low birthweight (under 5 pounds, 8 ounces).

How much activity do you really want during pregnancy?

Solid pregnant ladies need somewhere around 2½ long stretches of moderate-power oxygen consuming movement every week. Oxygen consuming exercises cause you to inhale quicker and profoundly and make your heart beat quicker. Moderate-power implies you're sufficiently dynamic to perspire and expand your pulse. Going for an energetic stroll is an illustration of moderate-power oxygen consuming movement. On the off chance that you can't talk ordinarily during a movement, you might be really buckling down. You don't need to do all 2½ hours without a moment's delay. All things being equal, split it up as the week progressed. For instance, complete 30 minutes of activity on most or throughout the days. On the off chance that this sounds like a great deal, split up the 30 minutes by accomplishing something dynamic for 10 minutes multiple times every day.

For what reason is actual work during pregnancy really great for you?

For sound pregnant ladies, customary activity can:

- Keep your psyche and body solid. Active work can help you feel significantly better and give you additional energy.
- It additionally makes your heart, lungs and veins solid and assists you with remaining fit.
- Assist you with putting on the perfect proportion of weight during pregnancy.
- Facilitate a few normal distresses of pregnancy, like obstruction, back torment and enlarging in your legs, lower legs and feet.

- Help you with directing tension and rest better. Stress is stress, strain or tension that you feel in light of things that occur in your life.
- Assist with diminishing your gamble of pregnancy inconveniences, like gestational diabetes and toxemia. Gestational diabetes is a sort of diabetes that can occur during pregnancy. It happens when your body has an excessive amount of sugar (called glucose) in the blood. Toxemia is a sort of hypertension a few ladies get after the twentieth seven day stretch of pregnancy or in the wake of conceiving an

offspring. These circumstances can expand your gamble of having inconveniences during pregnancy, like untimely birth (birth before 37 weeks of pregnancy).

- Assist with diminishing your gamble of having a caesarean birth (likewise called c-segment). Caesarean birth is a medical procedure wherein your child is brought into the world through a cut that your primary care physician makes in your midsection and uterus.

Set up your body for work and birth. Exercises, for example, pre-birth yoga and Pilates can assist you with working on breathing, contemplation and other quieting strategies that might end up being useful to you overseeing work torment. Customary activity can assist with giving you energy and solidarity to overcome work.

What sorts of exercises are protected during pregnancy?

On the off chance that you're sound and you practised before you got pregnant, proceeding with your exercises during pregnancy is generally protected. Check with your supplier certainly. For instance, on the off chance that you're a sprinter or a tennis player or you do different sorts of extraordinary activity, you might have the option to continue to do your exercises when you're pregnant. As your midsection gets greater later in pregnancy, you might have to switch a few exercises or straightforwardness around on your exercises. If your supplier says it's Acceptable for you to work out, pick exercises you appreciate. On the off chance that you didn't practice before you were pregnant, this present time is an extraordinary opportunity to begin. Converse with your supplier about safe exercises. Begin gradually and develop your wellness gradually. For instance, begin with 5 minutes of movement every day, and move gradually for as long as 30 minutes every day.

These exercises for the most part are protected during pregnancy:

Strolling: Going for an energetic stroll is an extraordinary exercise that doesn't strain your joints and muscles. On the off chance that you're new tB07SPFD4ZH

Swimming and water exercises: The water upholds the heaviness of your developing child and moving against the water assists keep your heart rating up. It's additionally kind to your joints and muscles. On the off chance that you have low back torment when you do different exercises, take a stab at swimming.

Riding an exercise bike: This is more secure than riding a customary bike during pregnancy. You're less inclined to tumble off an exercise bike than a customary bicycle, even as your midsection develops.

Yoga and Pilates classes: Tell your yoga or Pilates instructor that you're pregnant. The educator can help you change or keep away from represents that might be hazardous for pregnant ladies, like lying on your midsection or level on your back (after the principal trimester). A few exercise centres and public venues offer pre-birth yoga and Pilates classes only for pregnant ladies.

Low-influence heart stimulating exercise classes: During low-influence heart stimulating exercise, you generally have one foot on the ground or hardware. Instances of low-influence heart stimulating exercise incorporate strolling, riding an exercise bike and utilizing a circular machine. Low-influence heart stimulating exercise don't overburden your body that **high-influence heart stimulating exercise do:** During high-influence heart stimulating exercise, the two feet leave the ground simultaneously. Models incorporate running, working out with rope and doing bouncing jacks. Let your educator know that you're pregnant so they can assist you with adjusting your exercise, if necessary.

Strength preparing: Strength preparing can assist you with building muscle and make your bones solid. It's protected to work out with loads for however long they're not excessively weighty. Get some information about the amount you can lift. You don't have to have a place with an exercise center or own extraordinary hardware to be dynamic. You can stroll in a protected region or do practice recordings at home. Or on the other hand observe ways of being dynamic in your regular day to day existence, such as accomplishing yard work or using the stairwell rather than the lift.

Is actual work alright for every single pregnant lady?

No. For certain ladies, practice isn't protected during pregnancy. Your supplier can assist you with understanding whether exercise is alright for you. The accompanying circumstances might make it dangerous to practice during pregnancy:

Preterm work, draining from the vagina, or your water breaking (additionally called cracked layers).

Preterm work is work that occurs before 37 weeks of pregnancy. Draining from the vagina and having your water break might be indications of preterm work. Being pregnant with twins, trios or more (additionally called products) with other gamble factors for preterm work. On the off chance that you're pregnant with products, inquire as to whether it's safe for you to work out. Your supplier might ask you to avoid extraordinary or high-influence exercises, like running. You might have the option to do low-influence exercises, such as strolling, pre-birth yoga or swimming.

Cervical inadequacy or a cerclage. The cervix is the opening to the uterus (belly) and is at the highest point of the vagina. Cervical inadequacy (additionally called bumbling cervix) implies your cervix opens (enlarges) too soon during pregnancy, for the most part without torment or constrictions. Cervical deficiency can cause untimely birth and unsuccessful labor. On the off chance that you have cervical deficiency or a short cervix, your supplier might suggest cerclage. This is a fasten your supplier places in your cervix to assist with keeping it shut so your child isn't conceived too soon. A short cervix implies the length of your cervix (likewise called cervical length) is more limited than ordinary.

Gestational hypertension or toxemia. Gestational hypertension is hypertension during pregnancy.

It begins following 20 weeks of pregnancy and disappears after you conceive an offspring. Placenta previa following 26 weeks of pregnancy. This is the point at which the placenta lies exceptionally low in the uterus and covers all or part of the cervix. The placenta fills in your uterus and supplies the child with food and oxygen through the umbilical string. Placenta previa can cause weighty draining and different entanglements later in pregnancy.

Serious iron deficiency or certain heart or lung conditions. Iron deficiency is the point at which you need more solid red platelets to convey oxygen to the remainder of your body. On the off chance that you show at least a bit of kindness or lung condition, inquire as to whether it's protected to practice during pregnancy.

What sorts of exercises aren't protected during pregnancy?

Be cautious and check with your supplier while picking your exercises. During pregnancy, don't do:

- Any action that has a great deal of jerky, skipping developments that might make you fall, similar to horseback riding, downhill skiing, rough terrain cycling, tumbling or skating.

- Any game wherein you might be hit in the midsection, like ice hockey, boxing, soccer or b-ball.
- Any activity that makes you lie level on your back (after the principal trimester), like sit-ups. At the point when you lie on your back, your uterus comes down on an enormous vein that takes blood back to your heart. Lying on your back can cause your circulatory strain to drop and restrict the progression of blood to your child.
- Exercises that can make you hit the water with

extraordinary power, similar to water skiing, surfing or plunging.

- Skydiving or scuba plunging. Scuba plunging can prompt decompression affliction. This is when hazardous gas bubbles structure in your child's body.
- Practising at high elevation (over 6,000 feet), except if you inhabit a high height. The elevation is the level of something over the ground. For instance, on the off chance that you're at a high elevation, you're most likely in the mountains. Practising at high elevations during pregnancy can bring down

how much oxygen that arrives at your child.

- Exercises that might make your internal heat level too high, such as Bikram yoga (additionally called hot yoga) or practising outside on hot, sticky days. you can do yoga in a room where the temperature is set. It's undependable for pregnant ladies since it can cause hyperthermia, a condition that happens when your internal heat level gets excessively high. A few examinations recommend that investing an excess of energy in a sauna or hot tub might make your internal heat level excessively high and increment your gamble of having a child who has birth surrenders. To be protected, don't spend over 15 minutes all at once in a sauna or more than 10 all at once minutes in a hot tub.

Does pregnancy change how your body answers work out?

During pregnancy, your body changes in numerous ways. At the point when you're dynamic, you might see changes in your:

Balance: You might see that you lose your equilibrium all the more effectively during pregnancy.

Internal heat level: Your internal heat level is marginally higher during pregnancy, so you begin perspiring sooner than you did before pregnancy.

Relaxing: As your child creates and your body transforms, you really want more oxygen. Your developing midsection comes down on your stomach, a muscle that assists you with relaxing. You might try and discover yourself feeling winded now and again.

Energy: Your body's endeavouring to deal with your child, so you might have less energy during pregnancy.

Pulse: Your heart works harder and pulsates quicker during pregnancy to get oxygen to your child.

Joints: Your body makes a greater amount of certain chemicals during pregnancy. This can make the tissues that help your joints more loose. Attempt to stay away from any developments that might strain or damage your joints.

When would it be a good idea for you to quit working out? What are the admonition signs you ought to look for while working out? While you're by and large genuinely dynamic, hydrate and focus on your body and how you feel. Stop your movement and call your supplier on the off chance that you have any of these signs or side effects:

- Draining from the vagina or liquid spilling from the vagina
- Chest torment, quick heartbeat or inconvenience relaxing
- Feeling discombobulated or faint
- Cerebral pain
- Muscle shortcoming, inconvenience strolling, or torment or enlarging in your lower legs. Torment or expanding in your lower legs might be indications of profound vein apoplexy (additionally called DVT). DVT happens when a blood coagulation structures in a vein somewhere down in the body, for the most part in the lower leg or thigh. On the off

chance that untreated, it can cause serious medical conditions and even passing.

- Customary, excruciating constrictions. A constriction is the point at which the muscles of your uterus get tight and afterward unwind. Constrictions assist with pushing your child out of your uterus.
- Your child quits moving. This might be a side effect of stillbirth (when a child kicks the bucket in the belly following 20 weeks of pregnancy).

Getting ready for conveyance

Having another youngster can be pure joy, but it can moreover be likewise incapacitating and overwhelming. Especially during the infant stage, you might find once routine undertakings troublesome due to one or the other absence of time, absence of energy or both. Arrangement can take the action into life as a parent more straightforward.

Ways Of getting ready for Work (delivery)

Your body normally gets ready for work all alone, however there are a couple of things you can do to assist with bringing down your pressure.

Take birthing classes: Birthing classes can answer a ton of your inquiries concerning what will occur during work and conveyance. You will figure out how to manage constrictions and remain in charge, and you will rehearse these methodologies so you're prepared for conveyance. Most ladies take their introduction to the world help individual with them to classes so they can rehearse together. Classes are generally accessible at your neighbourhood emergency clinic or birthing focus, however your primary care physician can assist you with tracking down the right class for you. It's really smart to take classes a couple of months before your due date, as they can top off rapidly.

Take breastfeeding classes: On the off chance that you've never breastfed, breastfeeding classes are a significant piece of getting ready for a child. These classes show you appropriate knowledge on how to hold your child while taking care of the child, and know when your child is getting enough. You could then find breastfeeding classes through your emergency clinic or neighborhood support programs. Taking a breastfeeding class allows you an opportunity to meet a lactation breastfeeding mother who can assist a large number of you with conceiving an offspring.

Take nurturing classes: Nurturing classes can assist you with understanding the various stages your child will go through, how to protect your child, how to dress and change your child, and how to tell when your child is having a health related crisis.

Make a birth arrangement: A birth plan is a framework of what you need for your conveyance. This plan helps your primary care physician or maternity specialist, medical attendants, and support individuals figure out your own desires. You ought to discuss your arrangement with your help individual and your primary care physician or maternity specialist. Not exclusively will it assist them with grasping you, however it will likewise assist you with sorting out whether or not what you have as a primary concern is plausible and ok for yourself as well as your child.

Birth plans ought to be working archives: Be adaptable and open to change, as births don't frequently go precisely true to form.

Visit the emergency clinic: Knowing what's in store and what to do can assist you with feeling more great upon the arrival of the birth. Set up an arrangement for a visit through the emergency clinic. A medical caretaker or other emergency clinic staff will take you through where you will have your child and what you can expect while you're there. This will likewise assist you with sorting out what choices are accessible so you can design your introduction to the world.

Gather your pack: You will require supplies for both you and your child at the emergency clinic. Emergency clinics might have various principles about what they give out to mothers and what you should bring from home.Prepare

All the Child Stuff ,Before the child shows up you ought to have specific things bought, collected, and tried to ensure they work and you know how to utilize them. We're firm professors in the toning it down would be ideal way of thinking with regards to child gear. The main fundamentals are an appropriately introduced vehicle seat and a protected spot for child to rest like a bassinet or lodging. In the event that you intend to utilize different things like a newborn child swing or evolving tables, you'll need to collect those also. A few things you won't use until the child is greater, for example, an exersaucer, however to collect all that you can while have opportunity and willpower. This doesn't need to be viewed as a tremendous errand as many individuals find embellishing and outfitting a nursery pleasant. A few ladies have "settling" inclinations while pregnant, and this is the ideal spot to channel that energy. Having a finished nursery, a lot of occasionally suitable garments, diapers and wipes will give you inward feeling of harmony

Chapter 2

post natal consideration

Post pregnancy care (PNC) is the consideration given to the mother and her infant following the birth and for the initial a month and a half of life (Figure 1.1). This period denotes the foundation of another period of day to day life for ladies and their accomplices and the start of the long lasting wellbeing record for infants (or youngsters — a term frequently utilized by specialists, medical attendants and midwives).Why is compelling post pregnancy care so significant?

At the point when successful post pregnancy care can have the most effect on the wellbeing and life chances of moms and babies is in the early neonatal period, the time soon after the conveyance and through the initial seven days of life. Be that as it may, the entire of the neonatal period, from birth to the 28th day after the birth, is a period of expanded risk. Passings during the initial 28 days of children who were conceived alive is accounted for by all nations on the planet as the neonatal death rate (the quantity of children who kick the bucket in the initial 28 days) per 1,000 live births. Additionally, reports of maternal mortality incorporate passing's of ladies from inconveniences related with post pregnancy issues, not simply issues emerging during the birth. Both these rates are significant marks of the viability of post pregnancy care. So the principal motivation behind why you really want to zero in additional consideration and consideration on the post pregnancy period is that this is an exceptionally crucial time for the mother and her infant baby.This high gamble period is likewise the time with the most reduced inclusion of maternal and kid medical services . This is the second motivation behind why you really want to concentrate on post pregnancy care. Assuming all infants got high effect and financially savvy intercessions during the post pregnancy time frame, it is assessed that neonatal mortality could be diminished by between 10-27%. At the end of the day, high post pregnancy care inclusion could set aside to 60,000 infant lives

The post pregnancy time frame endures six to about two months, it is destined to start just after the child. During this period, the mother goes through numerous physical and close to home changes while figuring out how to really focus on her infant. Post pregnancy care includes:

Getting Sufficient Rest

Rest is significant for new moms who need to reconstruct their solidarity. To try not to get too worn out as another mother, you might have to rest when your child dozes

- keep your bed close to your bassinet's to make night feedings more straightforward
- permit another person to take care of the child with a container while you rest
- Eating Right

Getting appropriate nourishment

In the post pregnancy period is significant as a result of the progressions your body goes through during pregnancy and work. The weight that you acquired during pregnancy assists ensure you with having sufficient nourishment for bosom taking care of. Be that as it may, you really want to keep on eating a solid eating regimen after conveyance. Specialists suggest that bosom taking care of moms eat when they feel hungry. Put forth an extraordinary attempt to zero in on eating when you are really ravenous — not simply occupied or tired. keep away from high-fat snacks focus on eating low-fat food varieties that balance protein, starches, and products of the soil a lot of liquids.

Vaginal Consideration

New moms ought to make vaginal consideration a fundamental piece of their post pregnancy care. You might encounter vaginal irritation, on the off chance that you had a tear during conveyance pee issues like torment or a successive inclination to urinate discharge, including little blood clusters constrictions during the initial not many days after conveyance . Plan an exam with your primary care physician around a month and a half after conveyance to talk about side effects and get legitimate treatment. You ought to keep away from sex for four to about a month and a half after conveyance with the goal that your vagina has legitimate opportunity to recuperate.

The Important point

It's essential to remain as sound as conceivable during pregnancy and during the post pregnancy time frame. Keep steady over your medical services arrangements and adhere to your primary care physician's all's directions for the wellbeing and security of you and your child.

Chapter 3

Fundamental newborn children care

However much an infant gives pleasure, it brings an equivalent measure of liability too. Unexperienced parents generally go through an uneven ride while dealing with a child, which includes issues like absence of rest, mitigating the child, and taking care of. Be prepared for extraordinary changes in your way of life and recollect that the principal chuckle of your little one makes the battles you go through worth

Taking care of your child

Clean up (or utilize a hand sanitizer) prior to taking care of your child. Infants don't have serious areas of strength for a framework yet, so they're in danger for contamination. Ensure that each and every individual who handles your child has clean hands. At the point when our children are first given over to us, the vast majority of us don't exactly have the foggiest idea how to hold them yet. There is consistently that apprehension, particularly for first time guardians, that you're not holding this minuscule, little child accurately. What's more, you genuinely should deal with them with care. The neck of the kid is the most sensitive and while getting them you ought to hold your hand under their head. Since the child can't genuinely uphold their head without help from anyone else, the assignment is yours to ensure you are continuously holding the child right — one hand under the head and placing the other under the hips.

You additionally must watch out for the weaknesses on the top of the infant. Contacting these ought to be stayed away from however much as could reasonably be expected. To give the greatest possible level of insurance and encourage your child, consistently keep them hidden from everyone else. Never shake your infant, whether in play or in dissatisfaction. Shaking can cause draining in the cerebrum and even passing. In the event that you really want to wake your newborn child, don't do it by shaking — all things being equal, stimulate your child's feet or blow delicately on a cheek.

Holding and Alleviating

Holding, presumably one of the most pleasurable pieces of newborn child care, occurs during the delicate time in the principal hours and days after birth when guardians make a profound association with their baby. Actual closeness can advance a profound association. For newborn children, the connection adds to their close to home development, which additionally influences their advancement in different regions, like actual development. One more method for considering holding is "experiencing passionate feelings for" your child. Youngsters flourish from having a parent or other grown-up in their life who loves them genuinely. Start holding by supporting your child and delicately stroking the person in question in various examples. Both you and your assistant can in like manner take action to be "skin-to-skin," holding your baby against your own skin while dealing with or supporting. Children, particularly untimely children and those with clinical issues, may answer baby knead. Particular sorts of back rub might upgrade holding and help with newborn child development and improvement. Many books and recordings cover newborn child knead — ask your primary care physician for suggestions. Be cautious, but — children are not generally serious areas of strength for so grown-ups, so knead your child delicately. Babies for the most part love vocal sounds, like talking, chattering, singing, and cooing. Your child will most likely additionally love paying attention to music. Child clatters and melodic mobiles are other great ways of invigorating your baby's hearing. In the event that your little one is being particular, take a stab at singing, discussing verse and nursery rhymes, or perusing resoundingly as you influence or rock your child delicately in a seat. A few children can be surprisingly delicate to contact, light, or sound, and could frighten and cry effectively, rest not exactly expected, or dismiss their countenances when somebody talks or sings to them. Assuming that is the situation with your child, keep commotion and light levels low to direct. Wrapping up: which functions admirably for certain children during their initial not many weeks, is another alleviating procedure first-time guardians ought to learn. Legitimate wrapping up keeps a child's arms near the body while taking into consideration some development of the legs. Not in the least does wrapping up keep a child warm, however it appears to provide most babies with a feeling that everything is good and solace. Wrapping up likewise may assist with restricting the surprise reflex, which can wake a child.

This is the way to wrap up a child:

- Spread out the getting cover, with one corner collapsed over marginally.
- Lay the endearing face up on the sweeping with their head over the collapsed corner.
- Fold the left corner around the body and fold it underneath the rear of the child, going under the right arm.
- Bring the base corner up over the child's feet and pull it toward the head, collapsing the texture down if it draws near to the face. Be certain not to wrap it too firmly around the hips. Hips and knees ought to be marginally twisted and

ended up. Wrapping your child also firmly may expand the opportunity for hip dysplasia.

- Fold the right corner over the child, and fold it under the child's back on the left side, allowing just the neck and make a beeline for remain uncovered. To ensure your child isn't wrapped excessively close, ensure you can slip a hand between the sweeping and your child's chest, which will permit happy with relaxing. Ensure, in any case, that the sweeping isn't free to such an extent that it could become unravelled.

- Children ought not be wrapped up after they're 2 months old. At this age, a few children can turn over while wrapped up, which expands their gamble of unexpected baby passing condition (SIDS).

About Diapering

You'll most likely choose before you bring your child home whether you'll automating material dispensable diapers. Whichever you use, your little one will have filthy diapers around 10 times each day, or around 70 times each week. Before diapering your child, the happiness you include all provisions inside reach so you will not need to leave your baby unattended on the evolving table. You'll require:

- A flawless diaper
- hooks (if material prefold diapers are used)
- diaper treatment
- diaper wipes (or a compartment of warm water and an unblemished washcloth or cotton balls).

After every solid discharge or on thee other hand on the off chance that the diaper is wet, lay your child on their back and eliminate the filthy diaper. Utilize the water, cotton balls, and washcloth or the wipes to delicately clean your child's genital region off. While eliminating a kid's diaper, do so cautiously in light of the fact that openness to the air might make him pee. While cleaning a young lady, clear her base off of front to back to stay away from a urinary parcel contamination (UTI). To forestall or recuperate a rash, apply treatment. Continuously make sure to clean up completely in the wake of changing a diaper. Diaper rash is a typical concern. Ordinarily the rash is red and uneven and will disappear in a couple of days with steaming showers, some diaper cream, and a brief period out of the diaper. Most rashes happen in light of the fact that the child's skin is delicate and becomes aggravated by the wet or poopy diaper.

To forestall or recuperate diaper rash, attempt these tips:

- Change your child's diaper frequently, and at the earliest opportunity after solid discharges. Delicately spotless the region with gentle cleanser and water (wipes some of the time can be disturbing), then, at that point, apply an exceptionally thick layer of diaper rash or "obstruction" cream. Creams with zinc oxide are favoured in light of the fact that they structure an obstruction against dampness.

- On the off chance that you use material diapers, wash them in colour and aroma free cleansers.
- Let the child go undiapered for part of the day. This allows the skin an opportunity to let some circulation into.
- On the off chance that the diaper rash go on for over 3 days or is by all accounts deteriorating, call your

primary care physician — it very well might be brought about by a contagious contamination that requires a prescription.

Bathing Nuts and bolts

You ought to give your child a wipe shower until:

- the umbilical string tumbles off and the navel recovers absolutely (1 month)
- the circumcision recuperates (1 fourteen days)
- A shower a couple of times every week in the foremost year is fine. More continuous washing might be drying to the skin.

Have these things prepared prior to washing your child:

- a delicate, clean washcloth
- gentle, unscented child cleanser and cleanser
- a delicate brush to invigorate the child's scalp
- towels or covers
- a spotless diaper
- clean garments

Wipe showers. For a wipe shower, select a protected, level surface (like an evolving table, floor, or counter) in a warm room. Fill a sink, if close by, or bowl with warm (not hot!) water. Disrobe your child and enclose the person in question by a towel. Wipe your newborn child's eyes with a washcloth (or a spotless cotton ball) hosed with water just, beginning with one eye and clearing off of the internal corner to the external corner. Utilize a spotless corner of the washcloth or another cotton ball to wash the other eye. Clean your child's nose and ears with the sodden washcloth. Then, at that point, wet the material once more and, utilizing a little cleanser, clean up delicately and wipe it off.

Then, utilizing child cleanser, make a foam and delicately wash your child's head and flush. Utilizing a wet material and cleanser, delicately wash the remainder of the child, really focusing on wrinkles under the arms, behind the ears, around the neck, and in the genital region. Whenever you have washed those regions, ensure they are dry and afterward diaper and dress your child.

Tub showers: When your child is prepared for tub showers, the principal showers ought to be delicate and brief. On the off chance that the individual in question ends up being disturbed, return to wipe showers for possibly 14 days, then, at that point, attempt the shower once more.

Notwithstanding the provisions recorded above, add:

an infant kid tub with 2 to 3 creeps of warm — not hot! — water (to test the water temperature, feel the water with inside your elbow or wrist). A newborn child tub is a plastic tub that can fit in the bath; it's a superior size for children and makes washing more straightforward to make due. Disrobe your child and afterward place the person in question in the water right away, in a warm room, to forestall chills. Ensure the water in the tub is something like 2 to 3 inches down, and that the water is done running in the tub. Utilize one of your hands to help the head and the other hand to direct the child in feet-first. Talking delicately, gradually bring down your child up to the chest into the tub. Utilize a washcloth to clean up and hair. Delicately knead your child's scalp with the stack of your fingers or a delicate child hairbrush, including the region over the fontanelles (weaknesses) on the highest point of the head. At the point when you flush the cleanser or cleanser from your child's head, cup your hand across the temple so the bubbles run toward the sides and cleanser doesn't get into the eyes. Delicately wash the remainder of your child's body with water and a limited quantity of cleanser. All through the shower, consistently pour water delicately over your child's body so the individual in question doesn't get cold. After the shower, envelop your child by a towel right away, making a point to cover their head. Child towels with hoods are perfect for keeping a newly washed child warm. While washing your newborn child, never let the child be. On the off chance that you really want to leave the restroom, enclose the child by a towel and take the person in question with you.

Circumcision and Umbilical String Care

Following circumcision, the tip of the penis is typically covered with dressing covered with petrol jam to hold the injury back from adhering to the diaper. Delicately clean the tip off with warm water after a diaper change, then, at that point, apply petrol jam to the tip so it doesn't adhere to the diaper. Redness or disturbance of the penis ought to recuperate inside a couple of days, however on the off chance that the redness or enlarging increments or on the other hand if discharge filled rankles structure, contamination might be available and you ought to call your child's primary care physician right away.

Umbilical rope care in babies is additionally significant. A few specialists propose cleaning the region with scouring liquor until the rope stump evaporates and tumbles off, normally in 10 days to 3 weeks, yet others suggest letting the region be. Converse with your kid's primary care physician to see what the person likes. A baby's navel region ought not be lowered in water until the string stump tumbles off and the region is recuperated. Until it tumbles off, the string stump will change tone from yellow to brown or dark — this is typical. Call your PCP in the event that the navel region looks red or on the other hand assuming that a foul smell or release creates.

Taking care of and Burping Your Child

Whether taking care of your infant by bosom or a jug, you might be puzzled regarding how frequently to do as such. For the most part, it's suggested that infants be benefited from interest — at whatever point they appear to be eager. Your child might signal you by crying, placing fingers in their mouth, or making sucking commotions. An infant should be taken care of each and every 2 to 3 hours. Assuming you're breastfeeding, allow your child the opportunity to nurture around 10-15 minutes at each bosom. Assuming that you're recipe taking care of, your child will no doubt take around 2-3 ounces (60-90 millilitres) at each taking care of. A few babies might should be stirred at regular intervals to ensure they get enough to eat. Call your child's PCP assuming that you really want to wake your infant frequently or on the other hand on the off chance that your child doesn't appear to be keen on eating or sucking. In the event that you're recipe taking care of, you can without much of a stretch screen assuming your child is getting enough to eat, however on the off chance that you're breastfeeding, it tends to be somewhat trickier. In the event that your child appears to be fulfilled, produces around six wet diapers and a few stools per day, rests soundly, and is putting on weight routinely, then the individual is most likely eating enough. One more effective method for telling assuming your child is getting milk is to see in the event that your bosoms feel full prior to taking care of your child and less full subsequent to taking care of. Converse with your PCP assuming you have worries about your kid's development or taking care of timetable. Babies frequently swallow air during feedings, which can make them fastidious. To assist with forestalling this, burp your child frequently. Have a go at burping your child each 2-3 ounces (60-90 millilitres) in the event that you bottle-feed, and each time you switch bosoms assuming that you breastfeed. Assuming your child will in general be gassy, has gastroesophageal reflux, or appears to be particular during taking care of, have a go at burping your little one after each ounce during bottle-taking care of or like clockwork during breastfeeding.

Attempt these burping tips:

- Hold your child upstanding with their head on your shoulder. Support your child's head and back while delicately tapping the back with your other hand.
- Sit your child on your lap. Support your child's chest and head with one hand by supporting your child's jaw in the center of your hand and resting the impact point of your hand on your child's chest (be mindful so as to hold your child's jaw — not throat).

Utilize the other hand to delicately pat your child's back.

- Lay your endearing face down on your lap. Support your child's head, ensuring it's higher than their chest, and tenderly pat or rub their back.

In the event that your child doesn't burp following a couple of moments, change the child's situation and have a go at burping for an additional couple of moments prior to taking care of once more. Continuously burp your child while taking care of time is finished, then save that person in an upstanding situation for somewhere around 10-15 minutes to abstain from throwing up.

Resting Fundamentals

As another parent, you might be shocked to discover that your infant, who appears to require you all day long, really rests around 16 hours or more! Babies normally rest for times of 2-4 hours. Try not to anticipate that yours should stay asleep for the entire evening — the stomach related arrangement of children is little to the point that they need sustenance at regular intervals and ought to be stirred on the off chance that they haven't been taken care of for 4 hours (or on a more regular basis assuming that your PCP is worried about weight gain). When could you at any point anticipate that your child should stay asleep from sundown to sunset? Many children stay asleep from sundown to sunset (between 6-8 hours) at 90 days old enough, yet in the event that yours doesn't, it's anything but a reason to worry. Like grown-ups, children should foster their own rest examples and cycles, so in the event that your infant is putting on weight and seems solid, don't surrender on the off chance that the person hasn't stayed asleep from sundown to sunset at 90 days. It's essential to constantly put children on their backs to rest to decrease the gamble of SIDS (unexpected baby demise disorder). Other safe resting rehearses include: not utilizing covers, quilts, sheepskins, squishy toys, and cushions in the den or bassinet (these can choke out a child); and sharing a room (yet not a bed) with the guardians for the initial a half year to 1 year. Likewise make certain to substitute the place of your child's head from one night to another (first right, then, at that point, left, etc) to forestall the improvement of a level spot on one side of the head. Numerous infants have their days and evenings "stirred up." They will quite often be more conscious and alert around evening time, and more lethargic during the day. One method for aiding them is to downplay excitement around evening time. Keep the lights low, for example, by utilizing a nightlight. Hold talking and playing with your child for the daytime. At the point when your child awakens during the day, attempt to keep that person conscious somewhat longer by talking and playing. Despite the fact that you might have a restless outlook on dealing with an infant, in a couple of brief weeks you'll foster an everyday practice and be nurturing like an expert! Assuming you have various forms of feedback, request that your PCP suggest assets that can assist you and your child with becoming together.

www.ingramcontent.com/pod-product-compliance
Lightning Source LLC
LaVergne TN
LVHW041121150826
845673LV00007B/2152

* 9 7 9 8 3 5 9 1 4 1 8 0 2 *